GASTROESOPHAGEAL REFLUX DISEASE (GERD) COOKBOOK FOR BEGINNERS

Navigate GERD With Confidence: Proven Methods, Dietary Tips, And Holistic Approaches For Long-Term Relief And Restoring Digestive Health

DR. JACE ZAYDEN

Table of Contents

Copyright © 2024, Dr. Jace Zayden

All Rights Reserved

No part of this publication may be reproduced, distributed, or transmitted in any form or by any means, including photocopying, recording, or other electronic or mechanical methods, without the prior written permission of the publisher, except in the case of brief quotations embodied in critical reviews and certain other noncommercial uses permitted by copyright law.

DISCLAIMER

The information provided in the book is intended for general informational purposes only. The content of this book should not be considered a substitute for professional medical advice, diagnosis, or treatment.

Readers are advised to consult with a qualified healthcare professional for medical advice tailored to their individual circumstances.

The author has made every effort to ensure that the information in this book is accurate and up-to-date at the time of publication. However, medical knowledge is constantly evolving, and new research may emerge that could impact the information presented. The author disclaims any responsibility for any adverse effects or consequences resulting from the use of the information provided in this book.

References or mentions of individuals, products, websites, organizations, or other names within this book are for informational purposes only and do not constitute an endorsement. The author has no affiliations with, and makes no endorsements of, any third-party entities mentioned. Readers are encouraged to conduct their own research and exercise their judgment when considering any external resources or recommendations.

The author and the publisher shall have neither liability nor responsibility to any person or entity with respect to any loss, damage, or injury caused or alleged to be caused directly or indirectly by the information contained in this book. Any reliance on the information within this book is at the reader's own risk.

By reading this book, the reader acknowledges and agrees to the terms of this disclaimer. If the reader does not agree with these terms, they should not use the information provided in this book.

ABOUT THIS BOOK

This "Gastroesophageal Reflux Disease (GERD) Cookbook" is an essential reference for those who are confronted with the difficulties of GERD management. It provides a thorough examination of dietary selections that have the potential to substantially mitigate symptoms and improve general health. Commencing with a comprehensive "Introduction," this book furnishes readers with a comprehensive synopsis of gastroesophageal reflux disease (GERD) and establishes the context for why incorporating a mindful approach to nutrition is crucial in its management. "Understanding Gastroesophageal Reflux Disease (GERD)" provides readers with a more comprehensive understanding of the condition's complexities.

This book places significant emphasis on the examination of the "Importance of Diet in Managing GERD," underscoring the critical nature of dietary decisions in alleviating symptoms. The following sections provide practical recommendations on which foods to incorporate and which to exclude, in addition to enlightening "Cooking Techniques for GERD-Friendly Meals." The incorporation of specialized chapters containing "Breakfast Recipes," "Lunch Ideas," and "Dinner Recipes" that cater to individuals with GERD provides readers with a wide range of options that are suitable for their palates.

This book additionally discusses the frequently disregarded elements of nibbles, appetizers, desserts, and treats that are appropriate for indulging in while managing gastroesophageal reflux disease (GERD). It acknowledges the criticality of maintaining a balanced and gratifying diet. "Beverages for GERD Management" delves into an assortment of beverage alternatives, while "Meal Planning Strategies" provides readers with the necessary resources to incorporate these suggestions into their routines.

This book offers practical guidance on "Eating Out with GERD" and crucial "Lifestyle Changes for Better GERD Management," thereby presenting a comprehensive approach to effectively managing real-life situations. "Quick and Easy GERD-Friendly Recipes" accommodate chaotic schedules, guaranteeing that the management of gastroesophageal reflux disease (GERD) does not sacrifice practicality. This book demonstrates its dedication to providing readers with exhaustive knowledge by including a section titled "Frequently Asked Questions about GERD and Diet" and "Sample Meal Plans" that provide structured guidance and address common concerns, respectively.

The "Gastroesophageal Reflux Disease (GERD) Cookbook" serves as an indispensable resource for individuals in search of a sustainable and pleasurable method to uphold a lifestyle compatible with GERD, in addition to alleviation of symptoms associated with the condition. Through the integration of medical knowledge and pragmatic culinary recommendations, this book functions as a definitive resource for individuals desiring to assert authority over their gastroesophageal reflux disease (GERD) experience by making well-informed dietary decisions.

CHAPTER ONE

Introduction

Chronic gastroesophageal reflux disease (GERD) is distinguished by the retrograde movement of gastric acid into the esophagus, resulting in the manifestation of symptoms including regurgitation, chest pain, and indigestion. A critical component of GERD management is the adoption of a dietary regimen that is tailored to the condition. Individuals afflicted with gastroesophageal reflux disease (GERD) can experience notable amelioration of symptoms and enhancement of their overall quality of life through the implementation of a customized nutritional regimen.

Gaining Comprehension Of Gastroesophageal Reflux Disease (GERD):

Gastric reflux disease (GERD) is a multifaceted disorder caused by the attenuation of the lower esophageal sphincter (LES), the muscular barrier separating the stomach and esophagus. As a result of improper closure of the LES, gastric acid may reflux into the esophagus, causing inflammation and irritation. Prolonged exposure to acid can induce harm to the esophageal membrane, thereby precipitating the distressing symptoms that are characteristic of gastroesophageal reflux disease (GERD).

GERD is frequently associated with obesity, pregnancy, tobacco use, and specific dietary patterns. For effective management, it is critical to comprehend the triggers and underlying causes of gastroesophageal reflux disease (GERD). Although medications can alleviate symptoms, adjustments in lifestyle, particularly in the area of diet, are of paramount importance in mitigating the risk of symptom recurrence and complications.

Dietary Importance In The Management Of GERD:

The management of gastroesophageal reflux disease (GERD) is significantly influenced by diet, as specific substances have the potential to induce or mitigate symptoms. The primary objectives of a gastrointestinal (GERD)-friendly diet are to reduce acid secretion, facilitate healthy digestion, and impede the reflux of stomach contents into the esophagus. Individuals who have gastroesophageal reflux disease (GERD) can enhance their quality of life and alleviate the severity and frequency of their symptoms through the selection of nutritious foods.

A balanced diet can contribute to overall health and assist in addressing other factors associated with GERD, such as obesity, in addition to symptom management. It is essential to maintain a healthy weight to alleviate gastric pressure and decrease the risk of acid reflux.

Moreover, by addressing inflammation and promoting healing of the esophageal membrane, dietary modifications can aid in the long-term management of gastroesophageal reflux disease (GERD).

Foods To Incorporate Into A Diet Friendly To GERD:

A GERD-friendly diet consists of consuming foods that have a reduced likelihood of inducing acid reflux and encourages the maintenance of a well-balanced and digestively comfortable eating routine. The following are essential elements of a GERD-friendly diet:

1. Lean Protein Sources: When selecting lean protein sources, consider poultry, fish, and tofu. These proteins facilitate digestion and are less likely to stimulate acid production.

2. Non-Citrus Fruits: Although citrus fruits may worsen symptoms of gastroesophageal reflux disease (GERD), non-citrus fruits such as pears, avocados, and melons are generally well-tolerated and offer vital vitamins and minerals.

3. While the majority of vegetables are well-tolerated for individuals with gastroesophageal reflux disease (GERD), it is prudent to refrain from consuming those that are known to induce flatulence, such as garlic and onions.

Typically, vegetables are more tolerable when steamed or sautéed.

4. Opt for whole grains over refined grains, such as quinoa, oats, and brown rice. These foods are rich in fiber, which promotes healthy weight maintenance and assists digestion.

5. Low-Fat Dairy Products: To mitigate the potential for reflux, choose dairy products that are low in fat or fat-free. Additionally, probiotic yogurt may be advantageous for digestive health.

6. Due to its anti-inflammatory properties, ginger is suitable for inclusion in a diet that is favorable to gastroesophageal reflux disease. It has the potential to alleviate symptoms and relieve the digestive tract.

7. Herbs and Spices: Although specific spices, such as fennel, basil, and turmeric, may induce gastric reflux, others possess anti-inflammatory properties and are generally well-tolerated.

By integrating these food items into their dietary regimen, individuals diagnosed with gastroesophageal reflux disease (GERD) can establish a harmonious and nutritious nutritional scheme that promotes the management of symptoms and enhances general health.

Foods To Prevent To Alleviate GERD:

An equally critical understanding pertains to the foods that have the potential to worsen symptoms of gastroesophageal reflux disease (GERD) and ought to be restricted in quantity or completely avoided. Several frequent offenders include:

1. Citrus Fruits: Tomatoes, oranges, and grapefruits are acidic foods that may exacerbate symptoms associated with acid reflux.

2. The LES can become relaxed during a meal of fried and fatty foods, permitting gastric acid to reflux back into the esophagus. Restrict the consumption of fried foods, decadent desserts, and fatty types of meat.

3. Caffeine and Chocolate: Due to their ability to relax the lower esophageal sphincter (LES) and stimulate acid secretion, both caffeine and chocolate are potential triggers for GERD symptoms.

4. Spicy Foods: Hot sauces, chile, and pepper are examples of spices that can irritate the esophagus and exacerbate acid reflux.

5. Because onions and garlic are known to induce indigestion and can relax the lower esophageal sphincter (LES), they are not recommended for people with GERD.

6. Although frequently linked to digestive health benefits, mint can relax the LES and exacerbate GERD symptoms.

7. Carbonated Beverages: The expansion of carbonated drink bubbles within the stomach can induce reflux and elevate intra-esophageal pressure. Instead, it is recommended to consume still water or medicinal beverages.

In summary, adhering to a GERD-friendly diet is an essential component in the management of gastroesophageal reflux disease. Through knowledge of the condition, prioritization of nutritious food selections, and avoidance of triggers, individuals can substantially mitigate the daily burden of gastroesophageal reflux disease (GERD). By integrating this dietary strategy with supplementary lifestyle adjustments and, if required, medical interventions, individuals can gain agency over their gastroesophageal reflux disease (GERD) and foster sustained health.

CHAPTER TWO

A Dietary Guide To Symptom Management

Chronic gastroesophageal reflux disease (GERD) is characterized by the persistent reflux of gastric acid into the esophagus, resulting in symptoms such as discomfort and irritation. Although medication can aid in symptom management, dietary modifications are of the utmost importance in reducing reflux episodes. In addition to being a valuable resource, The GERD Cookbook offers directions on how to prepare dishes that are easy on the digestive system. The primary objective of this gastronomic manual is to improve the quality of life and mitigate symptoms of gastroesophageal reflux disease (GERD).

Techniques For Preparing GERD-Friendly Dishes

Implementing culinary methods that decrease the probability of inducing gastroesophageal reflux disease (GERD)-friendly dishes are necessary for meal preparation. Fry-free alternatives to frying include grilling, roasting, and steaming, which reduce the utilization of lipids and oils that may exacerbate acid reflux. Moreover, reducing the intake of fatty portions of meat in favor of lean proteins such as poultry and fish can provide an additional layer of protection against irritation.

Herbs and seasonings that impart flavor without inducing discomfort must be utilized. Basil, parsley, and ginger are highly recommended options due to their anti-inflammatory and digestive-enhancing properties. Additionally, limiting the consumption of citrus fruits, garlic, and scallions can help mitigate their adverse effects on the digestive system.

By substituting smaller, more frequent meals for three large ones daily, one can reduce the risk of acid reflux by averting gastric excess. Engaging in comprehensive chewing of food facilitates digestion by reducing the workload on the stomach, thereby aiding in the management of symptoms.

Recipes For Breakfast With GERD

Breakfast that is GERD-friendly is essential for establishing a favorable mood for the remainder of the day. Served alongside sliced bananas and a drizzle of honey, oatmeal prepared with almond milk is a nourishing and calming alternative. Incorporating non-citrus fruits, such as melon and berries, into a fruit smoothie along with yogurt or a non-dairy substitute, can offer a revitalizing and reflux-friendly initiation to the day. A veggie and egg white omelet with spinach, mushrooms, and tomatoes is a low-acid, high-nutrient alternative for individuals who favor savory breakfasts. To incorporate additional nutrients without worsening symptoms of gastroesophageal reflux disease (GERD), consider pairing it with whole-grain crostini or a small portion of brown rice.

Lunch Suggestions For GERD Patients

GERD patients may find lunch to be a particularly difficult meal, as it frequently occurs during the middle of the day, when symptoms may be at their peak. Including grilled chicken, cucumbers, cherry tomatoes, and a light vinaigrette in a quinoa salad is a nutritious and reflux-friendly selection that promotes balance. Soups composed of lean proteins and vegetables with low acidity can also be calming and rich in vital nutrients.

The flavorful and GERD-friendly fish tacos comprised of whole-grain tortillas, cabbage slaw, and a moderate avocado-based vinaigrette make for an excellent lunch option.

To preserve the digestive health of these dishes, it is critical to refrain from incorporating citrus fruits or piquant salsas into them.

Recipes For Dinners To Manage GERD
While nourishing the body and providing an opportunity to relax, dinner does not provoke GERD symptoms. Salmon prepared in this manner, accompanied by roasted sweet potatoes and steamed broccoli, is an easy-to-digest and nutrient-dense dinner option. The inclusion of whole cereals such as brown rice or quinoa can

increase satiety without overburdening the digestive system.

An alternative to traditional dinners, a stir-fry of vegetables, tofu, or lean protein that contains GERD-friendly ingredients and minimal oil is a flavorful and speedy option for supper.

Increasing the size of the portion and ensuring thorough digesting are additional practices that can aid indigestion.

Snacks And Appetizers To Alleviate GERD

GERD patients must consume nutritious snacks to maintain energy levels without aggravating symptoms. Fresh fruit slices accompanied by a fistful of unsalted nuts or a dollop of almond butter can serve as a gratifying and healthful refreshment. Vegetables accompanied by hummus or a dip made with Greek yogurt are a delectable and reflux-friendly alternative.

Consider a cucumber and avocado sushi roll or bruschetta with a tomato and basil garnish on whole-grain bread for an appetizer. These alternatives reduce the presence of acidic components while maintaining gratifying taste profiles.

In summary, the GERD Cookbook provides an all-encompassing manual on symptom management via conscientious dietary selections. By employing appropriate culinary methodologies, integrating GERD-friendly recipes into their breakfast, lunch, and dinner plans, and exercising discernment when selecting nibbles and canapés, individuals can savor a diverse and flavorsome dietary regimen while concurrently mitigating the inconveniences associated with GERD daily.

GERD-Friendly Indulgence

Managing gastrointestinal reflux disease (GERD) frequently necessitates a prudent adherence to a restricted diet. Those with gastroesophageal reflux disease (GERD) may find desserts and candies challenging to consume, as numerous traditional options can elicit symptoms of acid reflux. A thoughtfully curated cuisine for individuals with gastroesophageal reflux disease (GERD) allows them to partake in delectable sweets.

It is essential, when preparing delicacies for individuals with gastroesophageal reflux disease (GERD), to prioritize ingredients that have a reduced propensity to induce acid reflux. For an initial delicious treat, bananas, and melons are examples of fruits that are low in acidity. Desserts that integrate these fruits include fruit salads, smoothies, and even baked goods. Additionally, desserts composed entirely of whole grains and oat flour might be more digestible.

Desserts can be naturally sweetened with sugar alternatives such as honey, maple syrup, or agave nectar, which lack the acidic qualities characteristic of refined carbohydrates. By experimenting with these all-natural sweeteners, the potential for GERD symptoms to be triggered in confectionery is reduced, while the sweetness is maintained.

In addition, the substitution of almond or coconut flour for conventional wheat flour in baked goods can impart a delectable and earthy taste. Without causing distress, nuts and seeds, such as chia seeds and almonds, can be used to add texture and healthful fats to desserts.

Compared to milk chocolate, dark chocolate with a high cocoa content may be more GERD-friendly for individuals with a sugar tooth. Dark chocolate is a more refined option for confection aficionados due to its reduced sugar and calorie content.

Formulating desserts with reduced lipid content is crucial for the management of gastroesophageal reflux disease (GERD). This can be accomplished by selecting recipes that call for less butter or oil and utilizing lighter dairy alternatives such as almond or soy milk. These substitutes can be used to prepare baked products such as biscuits and muffins without sacrificing flavor.

A GERD-friendly dessert compendium should, in essence, feature an assortment of recipes that accommodate diverse palates and preferences. Striking an equilibrium between appetite satisfaction and GERD symptom management is crucial when it comes to chocolatey and fruity treats alike.

By exercising ingenuity and placing emphasis on ingredients that are low in acidity and fat, people with gastroesophageal reflux disease (GERD) can partake in delectable delicacies while safeguarding their digestive well-being.

CHAPTER THREE

Beverages For Gastroesophageal Reflux Disease (GERD) Management:

The selection of beverages is a crucial factor in the management of gastroesophageal reflux disease (GERD). While some beverages may alleviate symptoms, others may worsen them. A cookbook designed to accommodate gastroesophageal reflux disease (GERD) should encompass an exhaustive compilation of beverages that promote gastric well-being and mitigate the symptoms of acid reflux.

Water is an indispensable element in a repertoire of beverages that are suitable for individuals with GERD. Adequate hydration facilitates the neutralization of gastric acid and enhances digestive health as a whole. Herbal infusions, including ginger and chamomile, are calming alternatives that may facilitate digestion while preventing the onset of reflux. However, it is not advisable to consume peppermint tea due to its potential to relax the lower esophageal sphincter, which could exacerbate symptoms of gastroesophageal reflux disease (GERD).

Apple or pear juice, among other non-citrus juices, may be incorporated into the assortment of beverages that are suitable for individuals with GERD. By diluting these juices with water or selecting low-acid varieties, individuals with gastroesophageal reflux disease (GERD) can further benefit from their consumption. Alkaline-rich ingredients, such as spinach, almond milk, and avocados, can contribute to the nutritional value and digestive health benefits of smoothies.

Regarding intoxicating beverages, individuals with GERD should practice moderation. Beverages with lower acidity, such as vodka or gin blended with non-citrus liquids, maybe more tolerable.

Consuming wine with caution is advised, specifically red wine, due to the potential to induce reflux in certain individuals.

GERD patients are frequently discouraged from consuming coffee and traditional caffeinated beverages on account of their acidic nature and propensity to relax the lower esophageal sphincter. Conversely, herbal infusions or caffeine-free alternatives such as chicory coffee or herbal infusions can be enjoyed without compromising on flavor for those with GERD.

Additionally, a cookbook designed to cater to gastroesophageal reflux disease (GERD) should incorporate preparations for domestic beverages that support digestive well-being. For example, aloe vera juice, which is renowned for its calming attributes, can be blended with water and a small amount of honey to create a revitalizing concoction. Warm water or coconut milk made with a sprinkle of turmeric contains an anti-inflammatory agent that may assist in the relief of GERD symptoms.

In essence, when considering beverages to complement a GERD-friendly diet, water, herbal teas, and non-citrus juices should take precedence over those that are excessively acidic or caffeinated. Identifying alternatives that not only provide hydration but also promote overall digestive comfort is crucial.

Strategies For Meal Planning With GERD

The organization of meals is an essential component in the management of gastroesophageal reflux disease. An intelligently designed cookbook catering to gastroesophageal reflux disease (GERD) should offer meal planning approaches that prioritize the reduction of triggers and the enhancement of digestive comfort.

Portion control is an essential component of meal planning for gastroesophageal reflux disease (GERD). Elevated abdominal pressure resulting from overeating can heighten the likelihood of developing acid reflux. A reduction in the frequency and size of meals consumed daily can aid in symptom management by averting the occurrence of excessive gastric distention.

Selecting the appropriate varieties of sustenance is of equal urgency. Meal plans that are suitable for individuals with gastroesophageal reflux disease (GERD) should prioritize whole, unprocessed foods while restricting the consumption of highly acidic or rich options. Meals may incorporate lean sources of protein, such as poultry, fish, and tofu, to prevent excessive strain on the digestive system.

Except for high-acid vegetables such as tomatoes and scallions, GERD-friendly dishes can benefit from the flavor and nutrients added by an assortment of vegetables. Quinoa, brown rice, and oatmeal are all excellent whole-grain options that are rich in fiber and do not exacerbate acid reflux.

Certain trigger foods, including citrus fruits, tomatoes, chocolate, and piquant foods, should be restricted or avoided. Additionally, alcoholic beverages, caffeinated beverages, and carbonated beverages should be consumed in moderation, if at all.

A cookbook designed for individuals with gastroesophageal reflux disease (GERD) may provide innovative recipe options that replace these triggers with milder alternatives that are more tolerable to the digestive system.

Meal timing is an additional factor that GERD patients must consider. Two to three hours before bedtime, eating meals can help reduce the likelihood of experiencing nocturnal regurgitation. Furthermore, maintaining a vertical alignment both during and following meals can aid in the prevention of retrograde reflux of gastric contents into the esophagus.

A cookbook designed to accommodate gastroesophageal reflux disease (GERD) should feature meal plans and recipes that accommodate various dietary restrictions and personal preferences. By integrating a diverse range of dishes into one's diet while maintaining a focus on GERD-friendly principles, individuals can savor delectable and gratifying meals without jeopardizing their digestive well-being, from breakfast to dinner.

Tips And Tricks For Eating Out With GERD

Those with gastroesophageal reflux disease (GERD) who dine out must employ a calculated approach to navigate restaurant menus and select items that promote digestive health. A cookbook designed for individuals with gastroesophageal reflux disease (GERD) should provide practical advice and strategies for dining out in a manner that prevents the onset of acid reflux symptoms.

It is advisable, when perusing a restaurant menu, to prioritize items that are prepared via grilling, baking, or steaming as opposed to frying. Considering that fried and fatty foods have the potential to worsen symptoms of gastroesophageal reflux disease (GERD), it is prudent to choose preparation methods that reduce the amount of added lipids.

When dining out with gastroesophageal reflux disease, it is a practical strategy to request dish modifications.

Numerous dining establishments demonstrate a readiness to cater to dietary restrictions by reducing the amount of oil used in preparations, omitting acidic components, or providing alternatives for trigger foods. Effective communication with the server regarding particular dietary requirements can contribute to a dining experience that is more conducive to individuals with gastroesophageal reflux disease.

Additionally, selecting side dishes and appetizers with care can contribute to a meal that is GERD-friendly. Choosing broth-based soups, salads adorned with non-acidic dressings, or vegetable-based appetizers may present themselves as more secure substitutes than alternatives loaded with acidic or spicy components.

When dining out, portion control remains crucial for those with GERD. One potential strategy to mitigate the occurrence of reflux symptoms is to request a half portion of an entree or share it. Additionally, eating slowly, savoring each bite, and allowing the stomach sufficient time to process the food, is recommended.

By substituting still water or herbal infusions for carbonated beverages, one can enhance the ambiance of the dining experience. When considering the consumption of alcohol, it may be more tolerable to select less acidic alternatives such as white wine or clear spirits blended with non-citrus liquids.

A GERD-friendly dish guarantees the availability of a secure alternative in communal settings where food sharing is customary, such as buffets or potlucks. This practice not only assists individuals suffering from gastroesophageal reflux disease (GERD) but also enhances the understanding of their dietary requirements among acquaintances and relatives.

A cookbook designed to accommodate gastroesophageal reflux disease (GERD) should ultimately enable diners to make well-informed decisions. By utilizing information regarding trigger foods, culinary techniques, and effective communication strategies, people with gastroesophageal reflux disease (GERD) can dine at restaurants while maintaining their digestive health.

CHAPTER FOUR

An All-Inclusive Manual For Symptom Management Via Diet

Gastroesophageal Reflux Disease (GERD) is a persistent medical condition distinguished by the retrograde movement of gastric acid into the esophagus. This reflux results in both irritation and possible harm to the esophageal membrane. GERD is frequently treated with a combination of dietary modifications, lifestyle adjustments, and medication. An essential component of this methodology is the GERD Cookbook, which is specifically crafted to furnish individuals with delectable recipes that are also compatible with reflux. This article will examine fundamental principles associated with the GERD Cookbook, encompassing modifications to one's lifestyle, expedient and effortless recipes, illustrative meal plans, and frequently asked inquiries.

The management of gastroesophageal reflux disease (GERD) is not solely dependent on dietary adjustments; lifestyle modifications are crucial in mitigating symptoms. By making minor modifications, the frequency and intensity of reflux episodes can be drastically diminished. The following adjustments to one's lifestyle are suggested to improve GERD management:

1. Head Elevation: By elevating the head of the bed by 6 to 8 inches, one can counteract the retrograde movement of gastric acid into the esophagus during slumber, a mechanism facilitated by gravity.

2. Sustain a Healthy Body Weight: Excessive weight, particularly in the abdominal region, can impede gastric circulation and exacerbate acid reflux. It can be advantageous to lose weight by consuming a well-balanced diet and engaging in consistent physical activity.

3. Avoid Trigger Foods and Beverages: GERD symptoms may be triggered by specific foods and beverages. Spicy foods, citrus fruits, tomatoes, chocolate, caffeine, and alcohol are frequent

offenders. The primary objective of The GERD Cookbook is to reduce or eliminate these triggers.

4. Replace large meals with smaller, more frequent ones to reduce the strain on the lower esophageal sphincter (LES), which can exacerbate acid reflux. By consuming smaller meals more frequently, excessive gastric distension can be avoided.

5. Cessation of Smoking: The LES is weakened by smoking, which facilitates the passage of gastric acid into the esophagus. In addition to being advantageous for overall health, quitting smoking is a crucial component in the management of gastroesophageal reflux disease (GERD).

Simple And Rapid GERD-Compatible Recipes:

The primary objective of The GERD Cookbook is to simplify and elevate the experience of meal preparation while strictly adhering to guidelines that are conducive to reflux. The following are some uncomplicated recipes that emphasize ingredients recognized for their ability to alleviate acid reflux and calm the digestive tract:

1. A breakfast consisting of oats accompanied by almond milk and bananas is a gratifying and calming choice. Add banana slices on top and substitute almond milk for dairy in place of acidic milk.

A straightforward salad comprising grilled chicken, cucumber, leafy greens, and a delicate vinaigrette can serve as a gratifying and gastroesophageal reflux disease (GERD)-compatible midday meal.

Salmon, which is an oily fish abundant in omega-3 fatty acids renowned for their anti-inflammatory attributes, was baked with quinoa. When baked with quinoa, it becomes a heartburn-friendly and nutritious dinner option.

4. Tea made with turmeric and ginger Both turmeric and ginger possess anti-inflammatory properties. After a long day, a calming tea crafted

from these components could be the ideal beverage to sip.

5. Smoothie with Bananas and Berries: Consolidate ripe bananas, berries, and a sprinkling of yogurt to create a delectable and reflux-compatible smoothie that can be utilized as an expedient breakfast alternative or refreshment.

Meal Plans Illustrative Of GERD Relief: Establishing a meal plan that is both balanced and suitable for gastroesophageal reflux disease (GERD) is essential for improving symptom management. The following is an example of a day's worth of dishes that adhere to the GERD dietary guidelines:

• Oatmeal accompanied by sliced bananas and a dusting of chia seeds for breakfast.

• Water or herbal tea.

• Quinoa served as a side dish accompanied by a grilled chicken salad comprised of mixed greens, cherry tomatoes, and a mild olive oil vinaigrette.

• Greek yogurt flavored with honey and a fistful of hazelnuts as a snack.

Baked salmon served with sautéed broccoli and quinoa or brown rice for supper.

• A sliced melon or a small apple as an evening snack.

Frequent Questions Regarding Diet And GERD

1. Am I still able to consume coffee if I have gastroesophageal reflux disease (GERD)? • Although coffee may provoke symptoms in some people, a reduced overall intake or low-acid coffee may be a more manageable alternative.

2. Are there particular fruits that I ought to refrain from consuming?

• Citrus fruits, including grapefruits and oranges, are frequently problematic. It is safer to consume less acidic fruits, such as melons, avocados, and berries.

3. Is occasional consumption of piquant cuisines permissible?

• GERD symptoms may be aggravated by spicy foods. Nevertheless, some people may discover that mild seasonings such as turmeric and ginger are more tolerable.

4. Is it imperative to entirely abstain from consuming chocolate? • Although certain individuals may find chocolate intolerable, moderate quantities of dark chocolate may be tolerable. Continual monitoring of individual responses is vital.

5. How close should I be to nightfall before I cease eating?

• It is recommended to reduce nocturnal reflux by consuming a meal that is fully digested two to three hours before slumber. This promotes adequate digestion time before assuming a supine position.

The GERD Cookbook is, in summary, a valuable resource for those in search of dietary remedies to alleviate the symptoms of GERD. Individuals can enhance their overall quality of life and effectively manage gastroesophageal reflux disease (GERD) by adopting proactive measures such as implementing lifestyle modifications, using simplified recipes, adhering to sample meal plans, and consulting dietary FAQs. It is imperative to consistently seek the guidance of a healthcare professional for individualized recommendations that are tailored to one's specific health conditions and requirements.

Conclusion

In summary, the Gastroesophageal Reflux Disease (GERD) Cookbook functions as an invaluable resource for those who are confronted with the difficulties associated with GERD management via dietary decisions. In its capacity as an all-encompassing manual, it not only furnishes an extensive assortment of delectable recipes but also enables readers to form enlightened judgments regarding their dietary practices. The cookbook assumes a critical role in fostering digestive health by emphasizing foods that mitigate symptoms and circumvent triggers.

Furthermore, the GERD Cookbook underscores the significance of embracing a comprehensive strategy in the management of GERD, recognizing that dietary modifications in isolation might not be adequate. The text promotes the adoption of a healthy lifestyle, which encompasses stress management and consistent physical activity, in addition to dietary improvements.

The cookbook acknowledges the uniqueness of each individual's GERD experience and provides adaptable recommendations. It fosters a harmonious and pleasurable eating culture, preventing individuals from experiencing deprivation while following GERD-friendly recommendations.

In essence, the GERD Cookbook not only discusses the physiological components of GERD management but also cultivates a constructive and enduring outlook on a way of life that promotes holistic health. By being a pragmatic and intuitive resource, it enables individuals to assume responsibility for their well-being and derive pleasure from an extensive assortment of delectable meals that are suitable for those with gastroesophageal reflux disease.

THE END